The Keto Cookbook

50 + Keto Diet Recipes, Easy Low Carb Plan For A Healthy Lifestyle And Quick Weight Loss

Celine Cunningham

Table of Contents

Introduction 5

Breakfast Recipes 12

1. Breakfast Porridge................................ 12

2. Easy Granola 14

3. Almond Cereal................................... 15

4. Breakfast Bowl 16

5. Breakfast Bread 18

6. Breakfast Muffins............................... 20

Lunch 21

7. Bacon Wrapped Sausages......................... 21

8. Lunch Lobster Bisque............................ 23

9. Simple Halloumi Salad 26

10. Lunch Stew 27

11. Chicken And Shrimp 29

Side Dishes & Dinner Recipes 31

12. Summer Side Salad 31

13. Tomato And Bocconcini 33

14. Cucumber And Dates Salad 34

15. Easy Eggplant Salad........................... 35

16. Special Side Salad 37

17. Special Endives And Watercress Side Salad....... 38

18. Indian Side Salad 40

19.   Indian Mint Chutney..41

    Seafoods Recipes..43

20.   Irish Clams...43

21.   Seared Scallops And Roasted Grapes.......................45

22.   Oysters And Pico De Gallo....................................47

23.   Grilled Squid And Tasty Guacamole........................49

24.   Shrimp And Cauliflower Delight.............................51

25.   Salmon Stuffed With Shrimp.................................53

26.   Mustard Glazed Salmon.......................................55

27.   Incredible Salmon Dish..56

28.   Scallops And Fennel Sauce....................................58

    Poultry Recipes..60

29.   Tender Chicken Thighs..60

30.   Crusted Chicken..62

31.   Pepperoni Chicken Bake.......................................63

32.   Fried Chicken..65

33.   Chicken Calzone..66

34.   Mexican Chicken Soup...68

35.   Simple Chicken Stir Fry..69

36.   Spinach And Artichoke Chicken.............................71

37.   Chicken Meatloaf..72

    Meat Recipes..74

38.   Lamb Riblets And Tasty Mint Pesto........................74

39.   Lamb With Fennel And Figs...................................76

40.   Baked Veal And Cabbage......................................78

41.   Beef Bourguignon..79

42. Roasted Beef...81

43. Beef Stew...83

44. Pork Stew...85

45. Sausage Stew..87

46. Burgundy Beef Stew..89

Vegetable Recipes 91

47. Arugula And Broccoli Soup 91

48. Zucchini Cream..93

49. Zucchini And Avocado Soup..95

50. Swiss Chard Pie 97

51. Swiss Chard Salad 99

52. Green Salad 101

53. Catalan Style Greens 102

Dessert and Snacks Recipes..104

54. Coconut And Strawberry Delight.....................................104

55. Caramel Custard 105

56. Cookie Dough Balls 106

57. Ricotta Mousse...108

58. Dessert Granola..109

59. Peanut Butter And Chia Pudding 110

60. Pumpkin Custard 111

61. No Bake Cookies...112

Introduction

What is Keto Diet?

Keto diet (Ketogenic diet) this is a low-carb diet with a high percentage of fat in the diet, in which the body produces ketones in the liver and uses them as energy.

Initially the main most familiar and accessible source of energy for our body is glucose. When you eat something high in carbohydrates, our body processes them into glucose, which increases the blood sugar and for its stabilization and the distribution of glucose in the cells of the body, the pancreas produces insulin.

Glucose is the simplest molecule in our body that is converted and used as energy, so it will be chosen over any other source of energy.

Insulin is produced to process glucose in the blood by moving it throughout the body.

Since glucose is used as an energy source, your fats are not needed and therefore accumulate. Typically, in a normal, higher carbohydrate diet, the body will use glucose as the main form of energy. By reducing carbohydrate intake, the body is induced into a condition known as ketosis.

Ketosis is a natural condition of our body, which starts with a low content of glucose in the diet. With him, the body produces ketones, splitting fatty acids, to provide us with a sufficient level of energy, nutrition of brain cells and organs.

The main goal and ultimate goal of keto diets is to switch us to the state of ketosis. It is important to understand that it does not start with a lowcalorie

intake, but with a low carbohydrate content in the diet.

Our bodies are incredibly adaptive - as soon as they lack glucose, they easily switch to ketosis and begin to use fats as the main source of energy.

The optimal level of ketones and low blood sugar levels give us a lot of advantages: from a general improvement in health and a decrease in the percentage of subcutaneous fat, to an increase in mental concentration, energy level and vitality.

A keto-diet implies a high fat content, a moderate protein content and a very low carbohydrate content.

Nutrient intake should be about 70% fat, 25% protein and 5% carbohydrates.

What Keto Can Do For You

Keto has its origins in treating healthcare conditions such as epilepsy, type 2 diabetes, cardiovascular disease, metabolic syndrome, auto-brewery syndrome and high blood pressure but now has much wider application in weight control.

This diet, then, will take you above and beyond typical results and propel youinto a new realm of total body health. If you want to look and feel the best youpossibly can, all without sacrificing your love of delicious food, then this is thecookbook for you.

Why are people going on the ketogenic diet even if they don't have epilepsy? As the keto diet became a more popular alternative to fasting, people began noticing additional benefits, like weight loss. Here are the most reported benefits of the low-carb, high-fat diet:

Cutting out lots of carbs can lead to weight loss

Significantly restricting carbs causes the body to produce ketones, but it also prevents excess glucose from getting stored as body fat. Lots of people who go on the keto diet find that losing weight is much easier. This is especially true if your current diet is high in refined, simple carbs like white bread, pasta, and sugar. Carbs are not inherently evil - as we mentioned before, the body actually needs them - but refined carbs are not very nutritious and usually end up stored as fat. When you eliminate them, weight loss is more likely.

The diet improves energy levels

You probably are familiar with the sluggish feeling after eating a carb-heavy meal. That's because your body is working so hard to process the carbs. You get an initial burst of energy and then a crash. When you cut out those refined carbs and instead eat foods higher in fat, that fatigue goes away. Your blood sugar levels become more stabilized throughout the day instead of going on a rollercoaster. The high-fat diet also helps with mental energy, since the brain is especially fond of fats found in coconut oil and fatty fish.

Your skin and hair health improve

A lot of people who go on the keto diet report having healthier skin, hair, and even fingernails. Fat is a hydrating nutrient, and hair and skin love it. Hair becomes shinier, sleeker, and less brittle. Skin also becomes healthier and less dry, while cutting out inflammatory foods like sugar can help clear up acne.

The keto diet might prevent certain diseases

There isn't a ton of research into the keto diet's effect on disease, but early studies are intriguing. Heart disease is a top killer, especially in the United States, and the keto diet can help people maintain better blood pressure. A high body mass is linked to heart disease, so losing weight thanks to the keto diet can also protect a person from the disease. The keto diet's effect on the brain is also significant, and studies have shown that ketones might help prevent and even treat brain disorders like Alzheimer's.

The Keto Flu and how to avoid it.

Keto flu is not a virus that infects only those who decide to try a ketogenic diet. This is the body's response to carbohydrate restriction.

The most common symptoms of keto-flu are craving for sugar, dizziness, irritability, fog in the head and poor concentration, stomach pain, nausea, cramps, muscle soreness and insomnia.

To avoid this, follow these simple rules:

1. Drink more water (with a pinch of unrefined salt).

Hydration is vital, especially when you are on a ketogenic diet. If during a keto diet you do not drink enough water, you can easily dehydrate and experience side effects.

2. Supplement your diet with sodium, potassium and magnesium.

To get enough potassium, add avocados and leafy greens such as spinach to your diet. Add a little crude salt to each meal and to water to replenish sodium levels.

Magnesium is another important mineral that can significantly ease your transition to ketosis. Although you do not lose magnesium, while limiting carbohydrates, it is important to help you prevent and eliminate cramps, improve sleep quality and increase insulin sensitivity. Simply add pumpkin seeds, almonds and spinach to your diet.

3. Eat more fat.

To help your body adapt, eat more fat. Fat provides Acetyl-CoA liver

cells, which they can use to make ketones.

4. In the morning, do exercises with low intensity.

When you wake up, fill the bottle with water and a pinch of salt, and go for
a walk. The walk should be at a pace where you can easily talk without
gasping. It is desirable to walk about an hour.

As you continue walking, you should feel better and better and more and

more awake. This is a form of low intensity exercise that will help increase
fat burning, and you will not have to suffer from keto flu.

5. Relieve stress through meditation.

When you start a ketogenic diet, you may be tenser and more irritable

than usual. This is due to the fact that your cortisol levels are slightly

higher than usual.

To help reduce cortisol levels and improve overall well-being, it is best to

do daily meditation.

Every day, for 15 minutes, just sit silently, inhaling and exhaling slowly

and deeply.

The purpose of meditation is not to be thoughtless, so as not to be

distracted by the thought, but to concentrate on breathing. This is how you train your mind so that life is less stressful.

6. A good sleep is the key to success.

Another way to reduce stress levels is to ensure good sleep. Good sleep is especially important for ketogenic diets. Without this, cortisol levels will increase, which complicates keto-flu and keto-adaptation. Sleep at least 7-9 hours every night, and if you feel tired in the middle of the day, lie down for 30 minutes or meditate.

To fall asleep faster at night, turn off all lights (including the phone) at least 30 minutes before you go to bed. This will help you translate your mind from work mode to sleep mode.

Breakfast Recipes

1. __Breakfast Porridge__

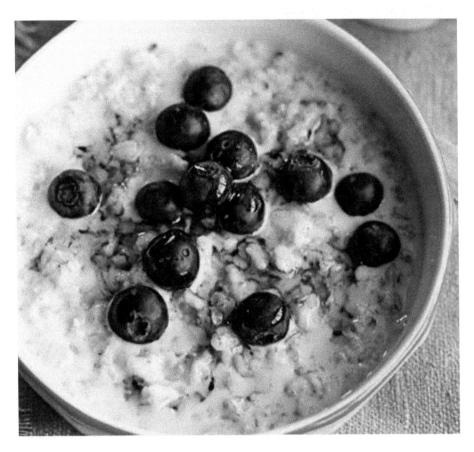

Preparation time: 5 minutes **Cooking time:** 10 minutes **Servings:** 1

Ingredients:

- 1 tsp. cinnamon powder
- A pinch of nutmeg
- ½ cup almonds, ground
- 1 tsp. stevia

- ¾ cup coconut cream
- A pinch of cardamom, ground
- A pinch of cloves, ground

Instructions:

1. Heat up a pan over medium heat, add coconut cream and heat up for a few minutes.

2. Add stevia and almonds and stir well for 5 minutes.

3. Add cloves, cardamom, nutmeg and cinnamon and stir well.

4. Transfer to a bowl and serve hot.

Nutrition: cal. 200, fat 12, fiber 4, carbs 8, protein 16

2. <u>Easy Granola</u>

Preparation time: 10 minutes **Cooking time:** 0 minutes **Servings:** 2

Ingredients:

- 2 tbsp. chocolate, chopped
- 7 strawberries, chopped
- A splash of lemon juice
- 2 tbsp. pecans, chopped

Instructions:

1. In a bowl, mix chocolate with strawberries, pecans and lemon

juice.

2. Stir and serve cold.

Nutrition: cal. 200, fat 5, fiber 4, carbs 7, protein 8

3. Almond Cereal

Preparation time: 5 minutes **Cooking time:** 0 minutes.

Servings: 1

Ingredients:

- 2 tbsp. almonds, chopped
- 2 tbsp. pepitas, roasted
- 1/3 cup coconut milk
- 1 tbsp. chia seeds
- 1/3 cup water
- A handful blueberries
- 1 small banana, chopped

Instructions:

1. In a bowl, mix chia seeds with coconut milk and leave aside for 5 minutes.

2. In your food processor, mix half of the pepitas with almonds and pulse them well.

3. Add this to chia seeds mix.

4. Also add the water and stir.

5. Top with the rest of the pepitas, banana pieces and blueberries and serve.

Nutrition: cal.200, fat 3, fiber 2, carbs 5, protein 4

4. Breakfast Bowl

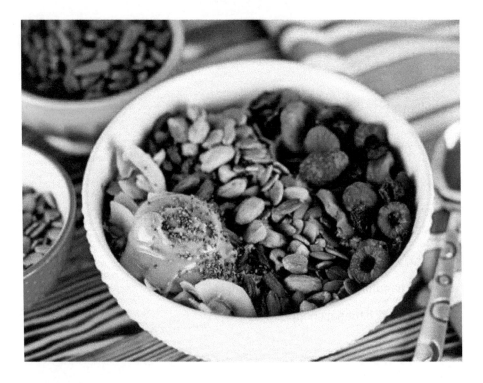

Preparation time: 5 minutes **Cooking time:** 0 minutes **Servings:** 1

Ingredients:

- 1 tsp. pecans, chopped
- 1 cup coconut milk
- 1 tsp. walnuts, chopped
- 1 tsp. pistachios, chopped
- 1 tsp. almonds, chopped
- 1 tsp. pine nuts, raw
- 1 tsp. sunflower seeds, raw
- 1 tsp. raw honey

- 1 tsp. pepitas, raw
- 2 tsp. raspberries

Instructions:

1. In a bowl, mix milk with honey and stir.

2. Add pecans, walnuts, almonds, pistachios, sunflower seeds,

pine nuts and pepitas.

3. Stir, top with raspberries and serve.

Nutrition: cal. 100, fat 2, fiber 4, carbs 5, protein 6

5. __Breakfast Bread__

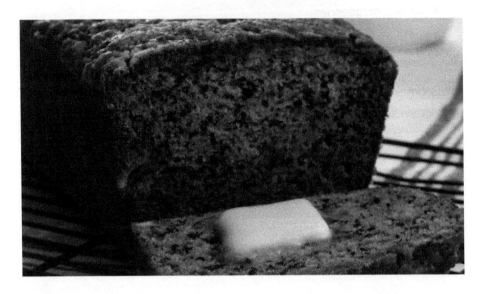

Preparation time: 10 minutes **Cooking time:** 3 minutes **Servings:** 4

Ingredients:

- ½ tsp. baking powder
- 1/3 cup almond flour
- 1 egg, whisked
- A pinch of salt
- 2 and ½ tbsp. coconut oil

Instructions:

1. Grease a mug with some of the oil.

2. In a bowl, mix the egg with flour, salt, oil and baking powder and stir.

3. Pour this into the mug and cook in your microwave for 3 minutes at a High temperature.

4. Leave the bread to cool down a bit, take out of the mug, slice and serve with a glass of almond milk for breakfast.

Nutrition: cal.132, fat 12, fiber 1, carbs 3, protein 4

6. Breakfast Muffins

Preparation time: 10 minutes **Cooking time:** 30 minutes **Servings:** 4

Ingredients:

- ½ cup almond milk
- 6 eggs
- 1 tbsp. coconut oil
- Salt and black pepper to the taste
- ¼ cup kale, chopped
- 8 prosciutto slices
- ¼ cup chives, chopped

Instructions:

1. In a bowl, mix eggs with salt, pepper, milk, chives and kale and stir well.

2. Grease a muffin tray with melted coconut oil, line with prosciutto slices, pour eggs mix, introduce in the oven and bake at 350 degrees F for 30 minutes.

3. Transfer muffins to a platter and serve for breakfast.

Nutrition: cal.140, fat 3, fiber 1, carbs 3, protein 10

Special Breakfast Bread

Lunch

7. Bacon Wrapped Sausages

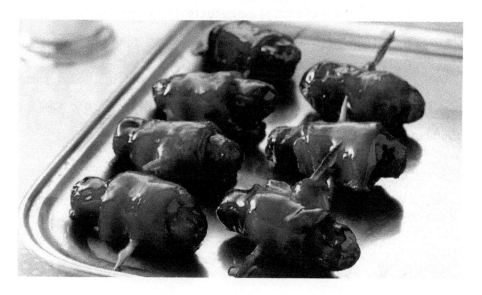

Preparation time: 10 minutes **Cooking time:** 30 minutes **Servings:** 4

Ingredients:

- 8 bacon strips
- 8 sausages
- 16 pepper jack cheese slices
- Salt and black pepper to the taste
- A pinch of garlic powder
- ½ tsp. sweet paprika
- 1 pinch of onion powder

Instructions:

1. Heat up your kitchen grill over medium heat, add sausages, cook for a few minutes on each side, transfer to a plate and leave them aside for a few minutes to cool down.

2. Cut a slit in the middle of each sausage to create pockets, stuff each with 2 cheese slices and season with salt, pepper, paprika, onion and garlic powder.

3. Wrap each stuffed sausage in a bacon strip, secure with toothpicks, place on a lined baking sheet, introduce in the oven at 400 degrees F and bake for 15 minutes.

4. Serve hot for lunch!

Nutrition: cal.500, fat 37, fiber 12, carbs 4, protein 40

8. <u>Lunch Lobster Bisque</u>

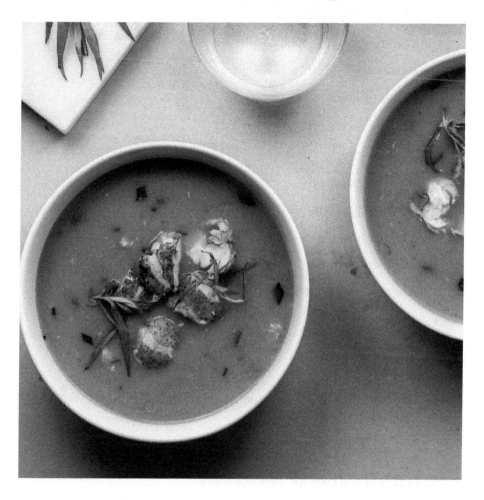

Preparation time: 10 minutes **Cooking time:** 1 hour **Servings:** 4

Ingredients:

- 4 garlic cloves, minced
- 1 small red onion, chopped
- 24 ounces lobster chunks, pre-cooked
- Salt and black pepper to the taste

- ½ cup tomato paste
- 2 carrots, finely chopped
- 4 celery stalks, chopped
- 1-quart seafood stock
- 1 tbsp. olive oil
- 1 cup heavy cream
- 3 bay leaves
- 1 tsp. thyme, dried
- 1 tsp. peppercorns
- 1 tsp. paprika
- 1 tsp. xanthan gum
- A handful parsley, chopped
- 1 tbsp. lemon juice

Instructions:

1. Heat up a pot with the oil over medium heat, add onion, stir

and cook for 4 minutes.

2. Add garlic, stir and cook for 1 minute more.

3. Add celery and carrot, stir and cook for 1 minute.

4. Add tomato paste and stock and stir everything.

5. Add bay leaves, salt, pepper, peppercorns, paprika, thyme and xanthan gum, stir and simmer over medium heat for 1 hour.

6. Discard bay leaves, add cream and bring to a simmer.

24

7. Blend using an immersion blender, add lobster chunks and cook for a few minutes more.

8. Add lemon juice, stir, divide into bowls and sprinkle parsley on top.

Nutrition: cal.200, fat 12, fiber 7, carbs 6, protein 12

9. <u>Simple Halloumi Salad</u>

Just gather all the ingredients you need and enjoy one of the best keto lunches!

Preparation time: 10 minutes **Cooking time:** 10 minutes **Servings:** 1

Ingredients:

- 3 ounces halloumi cheese, sliced
- 1 cucumber, sliced
- 1 ounce walnuts, chopped
- A drizzle of olive oil
- A handful baby arugula
- 5 cherry tomatoes, halved
- A splash of balsamic vinegar
- Salt and black pepper to the taste

Instructions:

1. Heat up your kitchen grill over medium high heat, add halloumi pieces, grill them for 5 minutes on each side and transfer to a plate.

2. In a bowl, mix tomatoes with cucumber, walnuts and arugula.

3. Add halloumi pieces on top, season everything with salt, pepper, drizzle the oil and the vinegar, toss to coat and serve.

Nutrition: cal.450, fat 43, fiber 5, carbs 4, protein 21

10. <u>Lunch Stew</u>

Preparation time: 10 minutes **Cooking time:** 3 hours and 30 minutes
Servings: 6

Ingredients:

- 8 tomatoes, chopped
- 5 pounds beef shanks
- 3 carrots, chopped
- 8 garlic cloves, minced
- 2 onions, chopped
- 2 cups water
- 1-quart chicken stock
- ¼ cup tomato sauce
- Salt and black pepper to the taste
- 2 tbsp. apple cider vinegar
- 3 bay leaves
- 3 tsp. red pepper, crushed
- 2 tsp. parsley, dried
- 2 tsp. basil, dried
- 2 tsp. garlic powder
- 2 tsp. onion powder
- A pinch of cayenne pepper

Instructions:

1. Heat up a pot over medium heat, add garlic, carrots and onions, stir and brown for a few minutes.

2. Heat up a pan over medium heat, add beef shank, brown for a few minutes on each side and take off heat.

3. Add stock over carrots, the water and the vinegar and stir.

4. Add tomatoes, tomato sauce, salt, pepper, cayenne pepper, crushed pepper, bay leaves, basil, parsley, onion powder and garlic powder and stir everything.

5. Add beef shanks, cover pot, bring to a simmer and cook for 3 hours.

6. Discard bay leaves, divide into bowls and serve.

Nutrition: cal.500, fat 22, fiber 4, carbs 6, protein 56

11.   **Chicken And Shrimp**

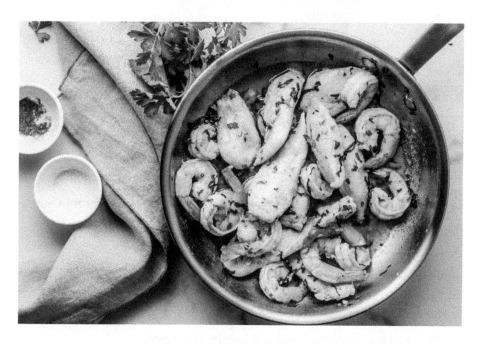

Preparation time: 10 minutes **Cooking time:** 20 minutes **Servings:** 2

Ingredients:

- 20 shrimp, raw, peeled and deveined
- 2 chicken breasts, boneless and skinless
- 2 handfuls spinach leaves
- ½ pound mushrooms, roughly chopped
- Salt and black pepper to the taste
- ¼ cup mayonnaise
- 2 tbsp. sriracha
- 2 tsp. lime juice
- 1 tbsp. coconut oil

- ½ tsp. red pepper, crushed
- 1 tsp. garlic powder
- ½ tsp. paprika
- ¼ tsp. xanthan gum
- 1 green onion stalk, chopped

Instructions:

1. Heat up a pan with the oil over medium high heat, add chicken breasts, season with salt, pepper, red pepper and garlic powder, cook for 8 minutes, flip and cook for 6 minutes more.

2. Add mushrooms, more salt and pepper and cook for a few minutes.

3. Heat up another pan over medium heat, add shrimp, sriracha, paprika, xanthan and mayo, stir and cook until shrimp turn pink.

4. Take off heat, add lime juice and stir everything.

5. Divide spinach on plates, divide chicken and mushroom, top with shrimp mix, garnish with green onions and serve.

Nutrition: cal.500, fat 34, fiber 10, carbs 3, protein 40

Side Dishes & Dinner Recipes

12.   <u>**Summer Side Salad**</u>

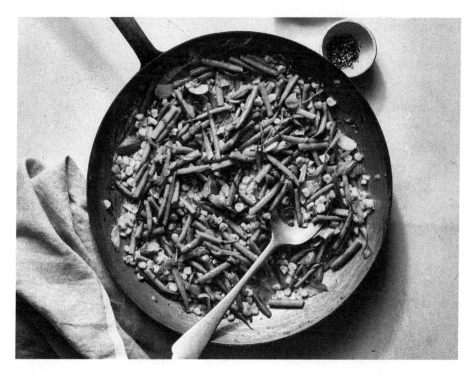

Preparation time: 10 minutes **Cooking time:** 5 minutes **Servings:** 6

Ingredients:

- ½ cup extra virgin olive oil
- 1 cucumber, chopped
- 2 baguettes, cut into small cubes
- 2 pints colored cherry tomatoes, cut in halves
- Salt and black pepper to the taste
- 1 red onion, chopped

- 3 tbsp. balsamic vinegar
- 1 garlic clove, minced
- 1 bunch basil, roughly chopped

Instructions:

1. In a bowl, mix bread cubes with half of the oil and toss to coat.

2. Heat up a pan over medium high heat, add bread, stir, toast for 10 minutes, take off heat, drain and leave aside for now.

3. In a bowl, mix vinegar with salt, pepper and the rest of the oil and whisk very well.

4. In a salad bowl mix cucumber with tomatoes, onion, garlic and bread.

5. Add vinegar dressing, toss to coat, sprinkle basil, add more salt and pepper if needed, toss to coat and serve.

Nutrition: cal.90, fat 0, fiber 2, carbs 2, protein 4

13. <u>Tomato And Bocconcini</u>

This salad goes really well with a grilled steak!

Preparation time: 6 minutes **Cooking time:** 0 minutes **Servings:** 4

Ingredients:

- 20 ounces tomatoes, cut in wedges
- 2 tbsp. extra virgin olive oil
- 1 and ½ tbsp. balsamic vinegar
- 1 tsp. stevia
- 1 garlic clove, finely minced
- 8 ounces baby bocconcini, drain and torn
- 1 cup basil leaves, roughly chopped
- Salt and black pepper to the taste

Instructions:

1. In a bowl, mix stevia with vinegar, garlic, oil, salt and pepper and

whisk very well.

2. In a salad bowl, mix bocconcini with tomato and basil.

3. Add dressing, toss to coat and serve right away as a keto side dish.

Nutrition: cal. 100, fat 2, fiber 2, carbs 1, protein 9

14. <u>Cucumber And Dates Salad</u>

Preparation time: 10 minutes **Cooking time:** 0 minutes **Servings:** 4

Ingredients:

- 2 English cucumbers, chopped
- 8 dates, pitted and sliced
- ¾ cup fennel, thinly sliced
- 2 tbsp. chives, finely chopped
- ½ cup walnuts, chopped
- 2 tbsp. lemon juice
- 4 tbsp. fruity olive oil
- Salt and black pepper to the taste

Instructions:

1. Put cucumber pieces on a paper towel, press well and transfer to a salad bowl.

2. Crush them a bit using a fork.

3. Add dates, fennel, chives and walnuts and stir gently.

4. Add salt, pepper to the taste, lemon juice and the oil, toss to coat and serve right away.

Nutrition: cal.80, fat 0.2, fiber 1, carbs 0.4, protein 5

15. <u>Easy Eggplant Salad</u>

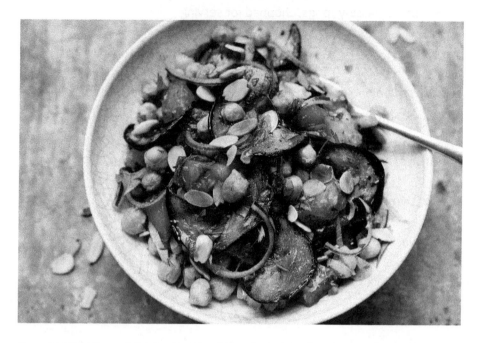

Preparation time: 10 minutes **Cooking time:** 10 minutes **Servings:** 4

Ingredients:

- 1 eggplant, sliced
- 1 red onion, sliced
- A drizzle of canola oil
- 1 avocado, pitted and chopped
- 1 tsp. mustard
- 1 tbsp. balsamic vinegar
- 1 tbsp. fresh oregano, chopped
- A drizzle of olive oil
- Salt and black pepper to the taste

- Zest from 1 lemon
- Some parsley sprigs, chopped for serving

Instructions:

1. Brush red onion slices and eggplant ones with a drizzle of canola oil, place them on heated kitchen grill and cook them until they become soft.

2. Transfer them to a cutting board, leave them to cool down, chop them

and put them in a bowl.

3. Add avocado and stir gently.

4. In a bowl, mix vinegar with mustard, oregano, olive oil, salt and pepper to the taste.

5. Add this to eggplant, avocado and onion mix, toss to coat, add lemon

zest and parsley on top and serve.

Nutrition: cal.120, fat 3, fiber 2, carbs 1, protein 8

16. Special Side Salad

Preparation time: 2 hours and 10 minutes **Cooking time:** 1 hour and 30

minutes **Servings:** 12

Ingredients:

- 1 garlic clove, crushed
- 6 eggplants
- 1 tsp. parsley, dried
- 1 tsp. oregano, dried
- ¼ tsp. basil, dried
- 3 tbsp. extra virgin olive oil
- 2 tbsp. stevia
- 1 tbsp. balsamic vinegar
- Salt and black pepper to the taste

Instructions:

1. Prick eggplants with a fork, arrange them on a baking sheet, introduce in the oven at 350 degrees F, bake for 1 hour and 30 minutes, take them out of the oven, leave them to cool down, peel, chop them and transfer to a salad bowl.

2. Add garlic, oil, parsley, stevia, oregano, basil, salt and pepper to the taste, toss to coat, keep in the fridge for 2 hours and then serve.

Nutrition: cal.150, fat 1, fiber 2, carbs 1, protein 8

17. Special Endives And Watercress Side Salad

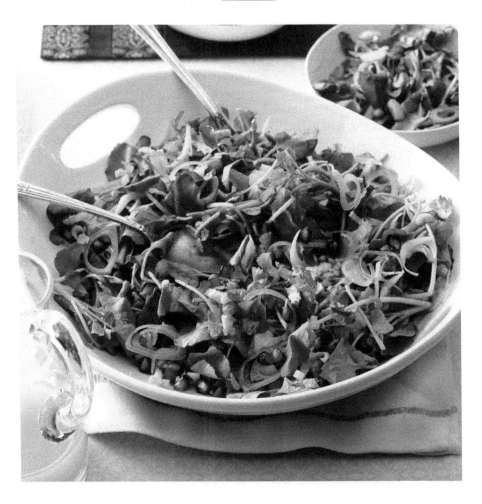

Preparation time: 10 minutes **Cooking time:** 5 minutes **Servings:** 4

Ingredients:

- 4 medium endives, roots and ends cut and thinly sliced crosswise
- 1 tbsp. lemon juice

- 1 shallot finely, chopped
- 1 tbsp. balsamic vinegar
- 2 tbsp. extra virgin olive oil
- 6 tbsp. heavy cream
- Salt and black pepper to the taste
- 4 ounces watercress, cut in medium springs
- 1 apple, thinly sliced
- 1 tbsp. chervil, chopped
- 1 tbsp. tarragon, chopped
- 1 tbsp. chives, chopped
- 1/3 cup almonds, chopped
- 1 tbsp. parsley, chopped

Instructions:

1. In a bowl, mix lemon juice with vinegar, salt and shallot, stir and leave a side for 10 minutes.

2. Add olive oil, pepper, stir and leave aside for another 2 minutes.

3. Put endives, apple, watercress, chives, tarragon, parsley and chervil in a salad bowl.

4. Add salt and pepper to the taste and toss to coat.

5. Add heavy cream and vinaigrette, stir gently and serve as a side dish

with almonds on top.

Nutrition: cal.200, fat 3, fiber 5, carbs 2, protein 10

18.   Indian Side Salad

Preparation time: 15 minutes **Cooking time:** 0 minutes **Servings:** 6

Ingredients:

- 3 carrots, finely grated
- 2 courgettes, finely sliced
- A bunch of radishes, finely sliced
- ½ red onion, chopped
- 6 mint leaves, roughly chopped
- *For the salad dressing:*
- 1 tsp. mustard
- 1 tbsp. homemade mayo
- 1 tbsp. balsamic vinegar
- 2 tbsp. extra virgin olive oil
- Salt and black pepper to the taste

Instructions:

1. In a bowl, mix mustard with mayo, vinegar, salt and pepper to the taste and stir well.

2. Add oil gradually and whisk everything. In a salad bowl, mix carrots with radishes, courgettes and mint leaves.

4. Add salad dressing, toss to coat and keep in the fridge until you serve it.

Nutrition: cal. 140, fat 1, fiber 2, carbs 1, protein 7

19.   <u>**Indian Mint Chutney**</u>

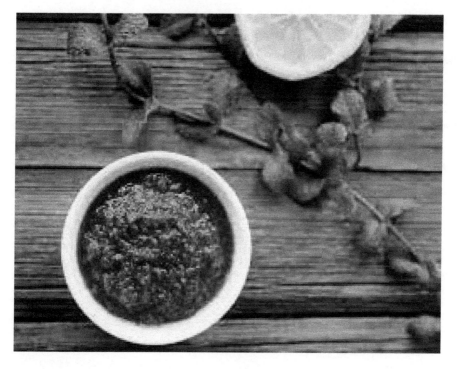

Preparation time: 10 minutes **Cooking time:** 0 minutes **Servings:** 8

Ingredients:

- 1 and ½ cup mint leaves
- 1 big bunch cilantro
- Salt and black pepper to the taste
- 1 green chili pepper, seedless
- 1 yellow onion, cut into medium chunks
- ¼ cup water
- 1 tbsp. tamarind juice

Instructions:

1. Put mint and coriander leaves in your food processor and blend them.

2. Add chili pepper, salt, black pepper, onion and tamarind paste and

blend again.

3. Add water, blend some more until you obtain cream, transfer to a bowl and serve as a side for a tasty keto steak.

Nutrition: cal. 100, fat 1, fiber 1, carbs 0.4, protein 6

Seafoods Recipes

20. **Irish Clams**

Preparation time: 10 minutes **Cooking time:** 10 minutes **Servings:** 4

Ingredients:

- 2 pounds clams, scrubbed
- 3 ounces pancetta
- 1 tbsp. olive oil
- 3 tbsp. ghee
- 2 garlic cloves, minced
- 1 bottle infused cider
- Salt and black pepper to the taste
- Juice of ½ lemon
- 1 small green apple, chopped
- 2 thyme springs, chopped

Instructions:

1. Heat up a pan with the oil over medium high heat, add

pancetta, brown for 3 minutes and reduce temperature to

medium.

2. Add ghee, garlic, salt, pepper and shallot, stir and cook for 3 minutes.

3. Increase heat again, add cider, stir well and cook for 1 minute.

4. Add clams and thyme, cover pan and simmer for 5 minutes.

5. Discard unopened clams, add lemon juice and apple pieces, stir and divide into bowls.

6. Serve hot.

Nutrition: cal.100, fat 2, fiber 1, carbs 1, protein 20

21. Seared Scallops And Roasted Grapes

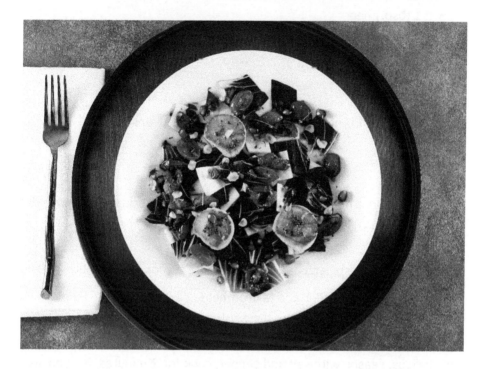

Preparation time: 5 minutes **Cooking time:** 10 minutes **Servings:** 4

Ingredients:

- 1 pound scallops
- 3 tbsp. olive oil
- 1 shallot, chopped
- 3 garlic cloves, minced
- 2 cups spinach
- 1 cup chicken stock
- 1 romanesco lettuce head
- 1 and ½ cups red grapes, cut in halves

- ¼ cup walnuts, toasted and chopped
- 1 tbsp. ghee
- Salt and black pepper to the taste

Instructions:

1. Put romanesco in your food processor, blend and transfer to a bowl.

2. Heat up a pan with 2 tbsp. oil over medium high heat, add shallot and garlic, stir and cook for 1 minute.

3. Add romanesco, spinach and 1 cup stock, stir, cook for 3 minutes, blend using an immersion blender and take off heat.

4. Heat up another pan with 1 tbsp. oil and the ghee over medium high heat, add scallops, season with salt and pepper, cook for 2 minutes, flip and sear for 1 minute more.

5. Divide romanesco mix on plates, add scallops on the side, top with walnuts and grapes and serve.

Nutrition: cal. 300, fat 12, fiber 2, carbs 6, protein 20

22.   Oysters And Pico De Gallo

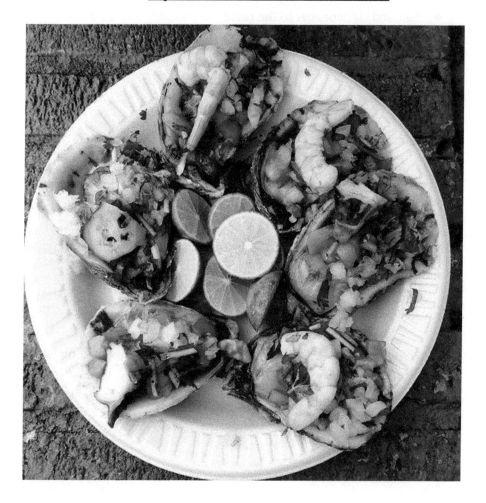

Preparation time: 10 minutes **Cooking time:** 10 minutes **Servings:** 6

Ingredients:

- 18 oysters, scrubbed
- A handful cilantro, chopped
- 2 tomatoes, chopped
- 1 jalapeno pepper, chopped

- ¼ cup red onion, finely chopped
- Salt and black pepper to the taste
- ½ cup Monterey Jack cheese, shredded
- 2 limes, cut into wedges
- Juice from 1 lime

Instructions:

1. In a bowl, mix onion with jalapeno, cilantro, tomatoes, salt, pepper and lime juice and stir well.

2. Place oysters on preheated grill over medium high heat, cover grill and cook for 7 minutes until they open.

3. Transfer opened oysters to a heatproof dish and discard unopened ones.

4. Top oysters with cheese and introduce in preheated broiler for 1 minute.

5. Arrange oysters on a platter, top each with tomatoes mix you've made earlier and serve with lime wedges on the side.

Nutrition: cal. 70, fat 2, fiber 0, carbs 1, protein 1

23. Grilled Squid And Tasty Guacamole

Preparation time: 10 minutes **Cooking time:** 10 minutes **Servings:** 2

Ingredients:

- 2 medium squids, tentacles separated and tubes scored lengthwise
- A drizzle of olive oil
- Juice from 1 lime
- Salt and black pepper to the taste
- *For the guacamole:*
- 2 avocados, pitted, peeled and chopped
- Some coriander springs, chopped
- 2 red chilies, chopped
- 1 tomato, chopped
- 1 red onion, chopped
- Juice from 2 limes

Instructions:

1. Season squid and squid tentacles with salt, pepper, drizzle some olive oil and massage well.

2. Place on preheated grill over medium high heat score side down and cook for 2 minutes.

3. Flip and cook for 2 minutes more and transfer to a bowl.

4. Add juice from 1 lime, toss to coat and keep warm.

5. Put avocado in a bowl and mash using a fork.

6. Add coriander, chilies, tomato, onion and juice from 2 limes and stir well everything.

7. Divide squid on plates, top with guacamole and serve.

Nutrition: cal.500, fat 43, fiber 6, carbs 7, protein 20

24. **Shrimp And Cauliflower Delight**

Preparation time: 10 minutes **Cooking time:** 15 minutes **Servings:** 2

Ingredients:

- 1 tbsp. ghee
- 1 cauliflower head, florets separated
- 1 pound shrimp, peeled and deveined
- ¼ cup coconut milk
- 8 ounces mushrooms, roughly chopped
- A pinch of red pepper flakes
- Salt and black pepper to the taste
- 2 garlic cloves, minced
- 4 bacon slices
- ½ cup beef stock
- 1 tbsp. parsley, finely chopped
- 1 tbsp. chives, chopped

Instructions:

1. Heat up a pan over medium high heat, add bacon, cook until

it's crispy, transfer to paper towels and leave aside.

2. Heat up another pan with 1 tbsp. bacon fat over medium

high heat, add shrimp, cook for 2 minutes on each side and transfer to a bowl.

3. Heat up the pan again over medium heat, add mushrooms, stir and cook for 3-4 minutes.

4. Add garlic, pepper flakes, stir and cook for 1 minute.

5. Add beef stock, salt, pepper and return shrimp to pan as well.

6. Stir, cook until everything thickens a bit, take off heat and keep

warm.

7. Meanwhile, put cauliflower in your food processor and mince it.

8. Place this into a heated pan over medium high heat, stir and cook for 5 minutes.

9. Add ghee and butter, stir and blend using an immersion blender.

10. Add salt and pepper to the taste, stir and divide into bowls.

11. Top with shrimp mix and serve with parsley and chives

sprinkled all over.

Nutrition: cal.245, fat 7, fiber 4, carbs 6, protein 20

25. <u>Salmon Stuffed With Shrimp</u>

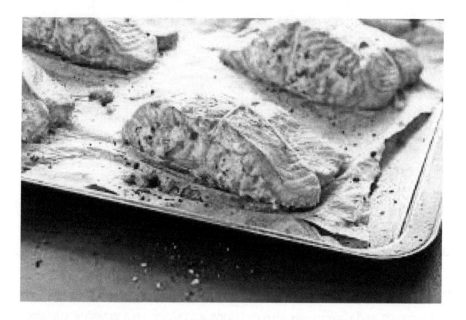

Preparation time: 10 minutes **Cooking time:** 25 minutes **Servings:** 2

Ingredients:

- 2 salmon fillets
- A drizzle of olive oil
- 5 ounces tiger shrimp, peeled, deveined and chopped
- 6 mushrooms, chopped
- 3 green onions, chopped
- 2 cups spinach
- ¼ cup macadamia nuts, toasted and chopped
- Salt and black pepper to the taste
- A pinch of nutmeg
- ¼ cup mayonnaise

Instructions:

1. Heat up a pan with the oil over medium high heat, add mushrooms, onions, salt and pepper, stir and cook for 4 minutes.

2. Add macadamia nuts, stir and cook for 2 minutes.

3. Add spinach, stir and cook for 1 minute.

4. Add shrimp, stir and cook for 1 minutes.

5. Take off heat, leave aside for a few minutes, add mayo and

nutmeg and stir well.

6. Make an incision lengthwise in each salmon fillet, sprinkle salt and pepper, divide spinach and shrimp mix into incisions and place on a working surface.

7. Heat up a pan with a drizzle of oil over medium high heat, add stuffed salmon, skin side down, cook for 1 minutes, reduce temperature, cover pan and cook for 8 minutes.

8. Broil for 3 minutes, divide between plates and serve.

Nutrition: cal.430, fat 30, fiber 3, carbs 7, protein 50

26. <u>Mustard Glazed Salmon</u>

Preparation time: 10 minutes **Cooking time:** 20 minutes **Servings:** 1

Ingredients:

- 1 big salmon fillet
- Salt and black pepper to the taste
- 2 tbsp. mustard
- 1 tbsp. coconut oil
- 1 tbsp. maple extract

Instructions:

1. In a bowl, mix maple extract with mustard and whisk well.

2. Season salmon with salt and pepper and brush salmon with half of the mustard mix

3. Heat up a pan with the oil over medium high heat, place salmon flesh side down and cook for 5 minutes.

4. Brush salmon with the rest of the mustard mix, transfer to a baking dish, introduce in the oven at 425 degrees F and bake for 15 minutes.

5. Serve with a tasty side salad.

Nutrition: cal.240, fat 7, fiber 1, carbs 5, protein 23

27. <u>Incredible Salmon Dish</u>

Preparation time: 10 minutes **Cooking time:** 15 minutes **Servings:** 4

Ingredients:

- 3 cups ice water
- 2 tsp. sriracha sauce
- 4 tsp. stevia
- 3 scallions, chopped
- Salt and black pepper to the taste
- 2 tsp. flaxseed oil
- 4 tsp. apple cider vinegar
- 3 tsp. avocado oil
- 4 medium salmon fillets
- 4 cups baby arugula
- 2 cups cabbage, finely chopped
- 1 and ½ tsp. Jamaican jerk seasoning
- ¼ cup pepitas, toasted
- 2 cups watermelon radish, julienned

Instructions:

1. Put ice water in a bowl, add scallions and leave aside.

2. In another bowl, mix sriracha sauce with stevia and stir well.

3. Transfer 2 tsp. of this mix to a bowl and mix with half of

the avocado oil, flaxseed oil, vinegar, salt and pepper and whisk well.

4. Sprinkle jerk seasoning over salmon, rub with sriracha and stevia mix and season with salt and pepper.

5. Heat up a pan with the rest of the avocado oil over medium high heat, add salmon, flesh side down, cook for 4 minutes, flip and cook for 4 minutes more and divide between plates.

6. In a bowl, mix radishes with cabbage and arugula.

7. Add salt, pepper, sriracha and vinegar mix and toss well.

8. Add this next to salmon fillets, drizzle the remaining sriracha

and stevia sauce all over and top with pepitas and drained

scallions.

Nutrition: cal. 160, fat 6, fiber 1, carbs 1, protein 12

28. Scallops And Fennel Sauce

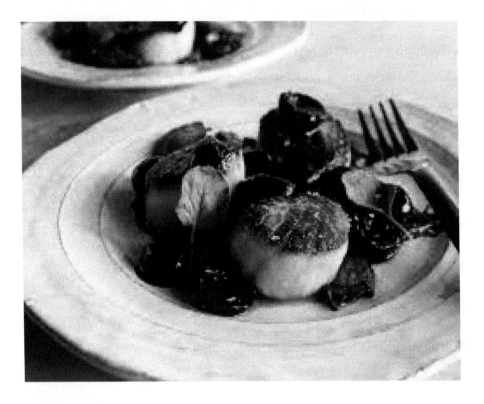

Preparation time: 10 minutes **Cooking time:** 10 minutes **Servings:** 2

Ingredients:

- 6 scallops
- 1 fennel, trimmed, leaves chopped and bulbs cut into wedges
- Juice of ½ lime
- 1 lime, cut into wedges
- Zest from 1 lime
- 1 egg yolk
- 3 tbsp. ghee, melted and heated up

- ½ tbsp. olive oil
- Salt and black pepper to the taste

Instructions:

1. Season scallops with salt and pepper, put in a bowl and mix with half of the lime juice and half of the zest and toss to coat.

2. In a bowl, mix egg yolk with some salt and pepper, the rest of the lime juice and the rest of the lime zest and whisk well.

3. Add melted ghee and stir very well.

4. Also add fennel leaves and stir.

5. Brush fennel wedges with oil, place on heated grill over medium high heat, cook for 2 minutes, flip and cook for 2 minutes more.

6. Add scallops on the grill, cook for 2 minutes, flip and cook for 2 minutes more.

7. Divide fennel and scallops on plates, drizzle fennel and ghee mix and serve with lime wedges on the side.

Nutrition: cal. 400, fat 24, fiber 4, carbs 12, protein 25

Poultry Recipes

29. <u>Tender Chicken Thighs</u>

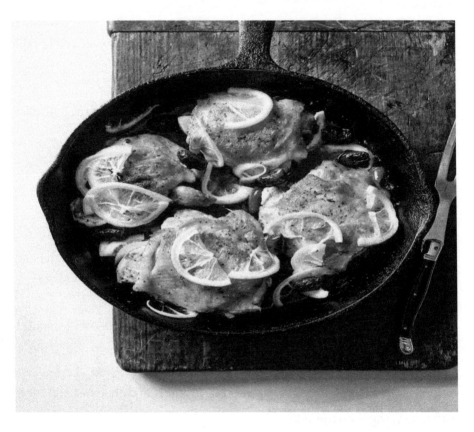

Preparation time: 10 minutes **Cooking time:** 45 minutes **Servings:** 4

Ingredients:

- 3 tbsp. ghee
- 8 ounces mushrooms, sliced
- 2 tbsp. gruyere cheese, grated
- Salt and black pepper to the taste

- 2 garlic cloves, minced
- 6 chicken thighs, skin and bone-in

Instructions:

1. Heat up a pan with 1 tbsp. ghee over medium heat, add chicken thighs, season with salt and pepper, cook for 3 minutes on each side and arrange them in a baking dish.

2. Heat up the pan again with the rest of the ghee over medium heat, add garlic, stir and cook for 1 minute.

3. Add mushrooms and stir well.

4. Add salt and pepper, stir and cook for 10 minutes.

5. Spoon these over chicken, sprinkle cheese, introduce in the oven at 350 degrees F and bake for 30 minutes.

6. Turn oven to broiler and broil everything for a couple more minutes.

7. Divide between plates and serve.

Nutrition: cal.340, fat 31, fiber 3, carbs 5, protein 64

30. Crusted Chicken

This is just perfect!

Preparation time: 10 minutes **Cooking time:** 20 minutes **Servings:** 4

Ingredients:

- 1 egg, whisked
- Salt and black pepper to the taste
- 3 tbsp. coconut oil
- 1 and ½ cups pecans, chopped
- 4 chicken breasts
- Salt and black pepper to the taste

Instructions:

1. Put pecans in a bowl and the whisked egg in another.

2. Season chicken, dip in egg and then in pecans.

3. Heat up a pan with the oil over medium high heat, add chicken and cook until it's brown on both sides.

4. Transfer chicken pieces to a baking sheet, introduce in the oven and bake at 350 degrees F for 10 minutes.

5. Divide between plates and serve.

Nutrition: cal. 320, fat 12, fiber 4, carbs 1, protein 30

31. <u>Pepperoni Chicken Bake</u>

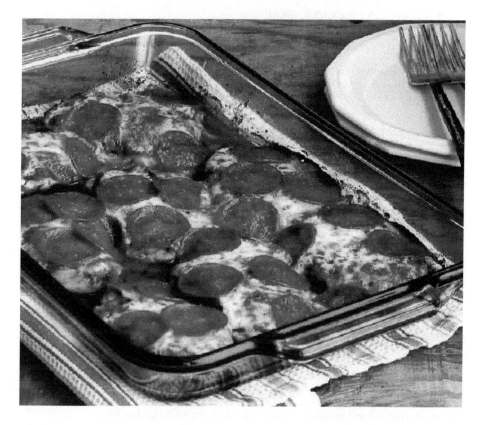

Preparation time: 10 minutes **Cooking time:** 55 minutes **Servings:** 6

Ingredients:

- 14 ounces low carb pizza sauce
- 1 tbsp. coconut oil
- 4 medium chicken breasts, skinless and boneless
- Salt and black pepper to the taste
- 1 tsp. oregano, dried
- 6 ounces mozzarella, sliced

63

- 1 tsp. garlic powder
- 2 ounces pepperoni, sliced

Instructions:

1. Put pizza sauce in a small pot, bring to a boil over medium heat, simmer for 20 minutes and take off heat.

2. In a bowl, mix chicken with salt, pepper, garlic powder and oregano and stir.

3. Heat up a pan with the coconut oil over medium high heat, add chicken pieces, cook for 2 minutes on each side and transfer them to a baking dish.

4. Add mozzarella slices on top, spread sauce, top with pepperoni slices, introduce in the oven at 400 degrees F and bake for 30 minutes.

5. Divide between plates and serve.

Nutrition: cal. 320, fat 10, fiber 6, carbs 3, protein 27

32. <u>**Fried Chicken**</u>

Preparation time: 24 hours **Cooking time:** 20 minutes **Servings:** 4

Ingredients:

- 3 chicken breasts, cut into strips
- 4 ounces pork rinds, crushed
- 2 cups coconut oil
- 16 ounces jarred pickle juice
- 2 eggs, whisked

Instructions:

1. In a bowl, mix chicken breast pieces with pickle juice, stir, cover and keep in the fridge for 24 hours.

2. Put eggs in a bowl and pork rinds in another one.

3. Dip chicken pieces in egg and then in rings and coat well.

4. Heat up a pan with the oil over medium high heat, add chicken pieces, fry them for 3 minutes on each side, transfer them to paper towels and drain grease.

5. Serve with a keto aioli sauce on the side.

Nutrition: cal. 260, fat 5, fiber 1, carbs 2, protein 20

33. <u>Chicken Calzone</u>

Preparation time: 10 minutes **Cooking time:** 1 hour **Servings:** 12

Ingredients:

- 2 eggs
- 1 keto pizza crust
- ½ cup parmesan, grated
- 1 pound chicken breasts, skinless, boneless and each sliced in halves
- ½ cup keto marinara sauce
- 1 tsp. Italian seasoning
- 1 tsp. onion powder
- 1 tsp. garlic powder
- Salt and black pepper to the taste
- ¼ cup flaxseed, ground
- 8 ounces provolone cheese

Instructions:

1. In a bowl, mix Italian seasoning with onion powder, garlic

powder, salt, pepper, flaxseed and parmesan and stir well.

2. In another bowl, mix eggs with a pinch of salt and pepper and

whisk well.

3. Dip chicken pieces in eggs and then in seasoning mix, place all

pieces on a lined baking sheet and bake in the oven at 350

degrees F for 30 minutes.

4. Put pizza crust dough on a lined baking sheet and spread half

of the provolone cheese on half

5. Take chicken out of the oven, chop and spread over provolone

cheese.

6. Add marinara sauce and then the rest of the cheese.

7. Cover all these with the other half of the dough and shape your

calzone.

8. Seal its edges, introduce in the oven at 350 degrees F and bake

for 20 minutes more.

9. Leave calzone to cool down before slicing and serving.

Nutrition: cal.340, fat 8, fiber 2, carbs 6, protein 20

34. __Mexican Chicken Soup__

Preparation time: 10 minutes **Cooking time:** 4 hours **Servings:** 6

Ingredients:

- 1 and ½ pounds chicken tights, skinless, boneless and cubed
- 15 ounces chicken stock
- 15 ounces canned chunky salsa
- 8 ounces Monterey jack

Instructions:

1. In your slow cooker, mix chicken with stock, salsa and cheese, stir,

cover and cook on High for 4 hours.

2. Uncover pot, stir soup, divide into bowls and serve.

Nutrition: cal.400, fat 22, fiber 3, carbs 6, protein 38

35. <u>Simple Chicken Stir Fry</u>

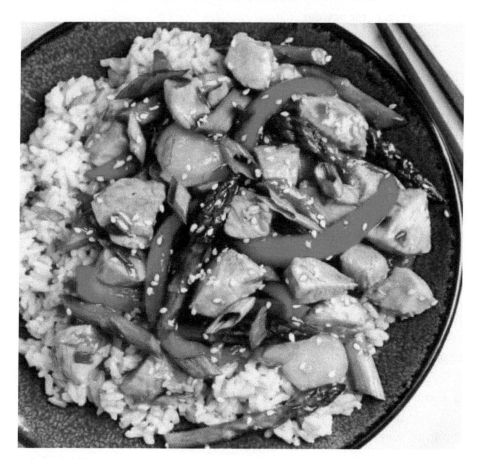

Preparation time: 10 minutes **Cooking time:** 12 minutes **Servings:** 2

Ingredients:

- 2 chicken thighs, skinless, boneless cut into thin strips
- 1 tbsp. sesame oil
- 1 tsp. red pepper flakes
- 1 tsp. onion powder
- 1 tbsp. ginger, grated

- ¼ cup tamari sauce
- ½ tsp. garlic powder
- ½ cup water
- 1 tbsp. stevia
- ½ tsp. xanthan gum
- ½ cup scallions, chopped
- 2 cups broccoli florets

Instructions:

1. Heat up a pan with the oil over medium high heat, add chicken and ginger, stir and cook for 3 minutes.

2. Add water, tamari sauce, onion powder, garlic powder, stevia, pepper flakes and xanthan gum, stir and cook for 5 minutes.

3. Add broccoli and scallions, stir, cook for 2 minutes more and divide between plates.

4. Serve hot.

Nutrition: cal. 210, fat 10, fiber 3, carbs 5, protein 20

36. Spinach And Artichoke Chicken

Preparation time: 10 minutes **Cooking time:** 50 minutes **Servings:** 4

Ingredients:

- 4 ounces cream cheese
- 4 chicken breasts
- 10 ounces canned artichoke hearts, chopped
- 10 ounces spinach
- ½ cup parmesan, grated
- 1 tbsp. dried onion
- 1 tbsp. garlic, dried
- Salt and black pepper to the taste
- 4 ounces mozzarella, shredded

Instructions:

1. Place chicken breasts on a lined baking sheet, season with salt and pepper, introduce in the oven at 400 degrees F and bake for 30 minutes.

2. In a bowl, mix artichokes with onion, cream cheese, parmesan, spinach, garlic, salt and pepper and stir.

3. Take chicken out of the oven, cut each piece in the middle, divide artichokes mix, sprinkle mozzarella, introduce in the oven at 400 degrees F and bake for 15 minutes more.

Nutrition: cal.450, fat 23, fiber 1, carbs 3, protein 39

37. __Chicken Meatloaf__

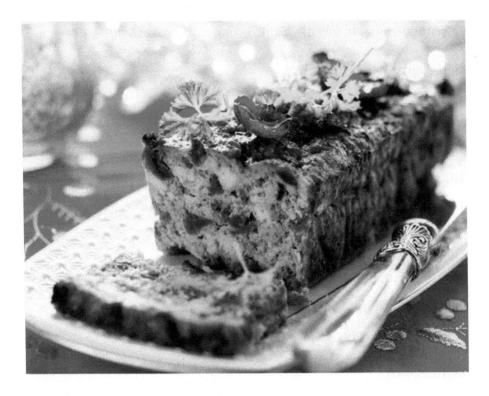

Preparation time: 10 minutes **Cooking time:** 40 minutes **Servings:** 8

Ingredients:

- 1 cup keto marinara sauce
- 2 pound chicken meat, ground
- 2 tbsp. parsley, chopped
- 4 garlic cloves, minced
- 2 tsp. onion powder
- 2 tsp. Italian seasoning
- Salt and black pepper to the taste

For the filling:

- ½ cup ricotta cheese
- 1 cup parmesan, grated
- 1 cup mozzarella, shredded
- 2 tsp. chives, chopped
- 2 tbsp. parsley, chopped
- 1 garlic clove, minced

Instructions:

1. In a bowl, mix chicken with half of the marinara sauce, salt, pepper, Italian seasoning, 4 garlic cloves, onion powder and 2 tbsp. parsley and stir well.

2. In another bowl, mix ricotta with half of the parmesan, half of the mozzarella, chives, 1 garlic clove, salt, pepper and 2 tbsp. parsley and stir well.

3. Put half of the chicken mix into a loaf pan and spread evenly.

4. Add cheese filling and also spread.

5. Top with the rest of the meat and spread again.

6. Introduce meatloaf in the oven at 400 degrees F and bake for 20 minutes.

7. Take meatloaf out of the oven, spread the rest of the marinara sauce, the rest of the parmesan and mozzarella and bake for 20 minutes more.

8. Leave meatloaf to cool down, slice, divide between plates and serve.

Nutrition: cal.273, fat 14, fiber 1, carbs 4, protein 28

Meat Recipes

38. <u>Lamb Riblets And Tasty Mint Pesto</u>

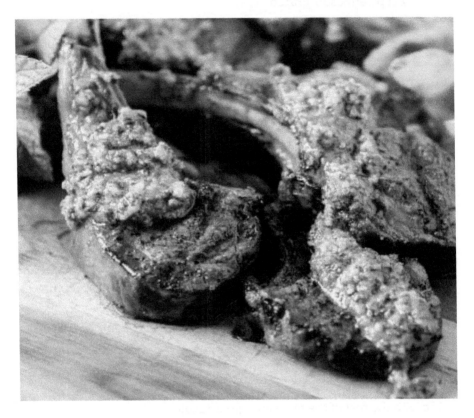

Preparation time: 1 hour **Cooking time:** 2 hours **Servings:** 4

Ingredients:

- 1 cup parsley
- 1 cup mint
- 1 small yellow onion, roughly chopped
- 1/3 cup pistachios
- 1 tsp. lemon zest

- 5 tbsp. avocado oil
- Salt to the taste
- 2 pounds lamb riblets
- ½ onion, chopped
- 5 garlic cloves, minced
- Juice from 1 orange

Instructions:

1. In your food processor, mix parsley with mint, 1 small onion, pistachios, lemon zest, salt and avocado oil and blend very well.

2. Rub lamb with this mix, place in a bowl, cover and leave in the fridge for 1 hour.

3. Transfer lamb to a baking dish, add garlic and ½ onion to the dish as well, drizzle orange juice and bake in the oven at 250 degrees F for 2 hours.

4. Divide between plates and serve.

Nutrition: cal. 200, fat 4, fiber 1, carbs 5, protein 7

39. **<u>Lamb With Fennel And Figs</u>**

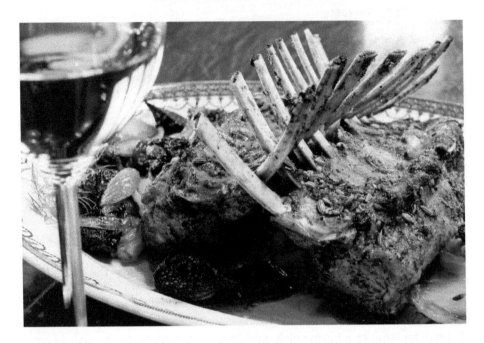

Preparation time: 10 minutes **Cooking time:** 40 minutes **Servings:** 4

Ingredients:

- 12 ounces lamb racks
- 2 fennel bulbs, sliced
- Salt and black pepper to the taste
- 2 tbsp. olive oil
- 4 figs, cut in halves
- 1/8 cup apple cider vinegar
- 1 tbsp. swerve

Instructions:

1. In a bowl, mix fennel with figs, vinegar, swerve and oil, toss to

coat well and transfer to a baking dish.

2. Season with salt and pepper, introduce in the oven at 400

degrees F and bake for 15 minutes.

3. Season lamb with salt and pepper, place into a heated pan over

medium high heat and cook for a couple of minutes.

4. Add lamb to the baking dish with the fennel and figs, introduce

in the oven and bake for 20 minutes more.

5. Divide everything between plates and serve.

Nutrition: cal. 230, fat 3, fiber 3, carbs 5, protein 10

40. **Baked Veal And Cabbage**

Preparation time: 10 minutes **Cooking time:** 40 minutes **Servings:** 4

Ingredients:

- 17 ounces veal, cut into cubes
- 1 cabbage, shredded
- Salt and black pepper to the taste
- 3.4 ounces ham, roughly chopped
- 1 small yellow onion, chopped
- 2 garlic cloves, minced
- 1 tbsp. ghee
- ½ cup parmesan, grated
- ½ cup sour cream

Instructions:

1. Heat up a pot with the ghee over medium high heat, add onion, stir and cook for 2 minutes.

2. Add garlic, stir and cook for 1 minute more.

3. Add ham and veal, stir and cook until they brown a bit.

4. Add cabbage, stir and cook until it softens and the meat is tender.

5. Add cream, salt, pepper and cheese, stir gently, introduce in the oven at 350 degrees F and bake for 20 minutes.

Nutrition: cal.230, fat 7, fiber 4, carbs 6, protein 29

41. **Beef Bourguignon**

Preparation time: 3 hours and 10 minutes **Cooking time:** 5 hours and 15 minutes **Servings:** 8

Ingredients:

- 3 tbsp. olive oil
- 2 tbsp. onion, chopped
- 1 tbsp. parsley flakes
- 1 and ½ cups red wine
- 1 tsp. thyme, dried
- Salt and black pepper to the taste
- 1 bay leaf
- 1/3 cup almond flour
- 4 pounds beef, cubed
- 24 small white onions
- 8 bacon slices, chopped
- 2 garlic cloves, minced
- 1 pound mushrooms, roughly chopped

Instructions:

1. In a bowl, mix wine with olive oil, minced onion, thyme,

parsley, salt, pepper and bay leaf and whisk well.

2. Add beef cubes, stir and leave aside for 3 hours.

3. Drain meat and reserve 1 cup of marinade.

4. Add flour over meat and toss to coat.

5. Heat up a pan over medium high heat, add bacon, stir and cook until it browns a bit.

6. Add onions, stir and cook for 3 minutes more.

7. Add garlic, stir, cook for 1 minute and transfer everything to a slow cooker.

8. Also add meat to the slow cooker and stir.

9. Heat up the pan with the bacon fat over medium high heat, add mushrooms and white onions, stir and sauté them for a couple of minutes.

10. Add these to the slow cooker as well, also add reserved marinade, some salt and pepper, cover and cook on High for 5 hours.

11. Divide between plates and serve.

Nutrition: cal.435, fat 16, fiber 1, carbs 7, protein 45

42. __Roasted Beef__

Preparation time: 10 minutes **Cooking time:** 8 hours **Servings:** 8

Ingredients:

- 5 pounds beef roast
- Salt and black pepper to the taste
- ½ tsp. celery salt
- 2 tsp. chili powder
- 1 tbsp. avocado oil
- 1 tbsp. sweet paprika
- A pinch of cayenne pepper
- ½ tsp. garlic powder
- ½ cup beef stock
- 1 tbsp. garlic, minced
- ¼ tsp. dry mustard

Instructions:

1. Heat up a pan with the oil over medium high heat, add beef

roast and brown it on all sides.

2. In a bowl, mix paprika with chili powder, celery salt, salt,

pepper, cayenne, garlic powder and mustard powder and stir.

3. Add roast, rub well and transfer it to a Crockpot.

4. Add beef stock and garlic over roast and cook on Low for 8

hours.

5. Transfer beef to a cutting board, leave it to cool down a bit, slice and divide between plates.

6. Strain juices from the pot, drizzle over meat and serve.

Nutrition: cal. 180, fat 5, fiber 1, carbs 5, protein 25

43. **Beef Stew**

Preparation time: 10 minutes **Cooking time:** 4 hours and 10 minutes
Servings:

4

Ingredients:

- 8 ounces pancetta, chopped
- 4 pounds beef, cubed
- 4 garlic cloves, minced
- 2 brown onions, chopped
- 2 tbsp. olive oil
- 4 tbsp. red vinegar
- 4 cups beef stock
- 2 tbsp. tomato paste
- 2 cinnamon sticks
- 3 lemon peel strips
- A handful parsley, chopped
- 4 thyme springs
- 2 tbsp. ghee
- Salt and black pepper to the taste

Instructions:

1. Heat up a pan with the oil over medium high heat, add

pancetta, onion and garlic, stir and cook for 5 minutes.

Add beef, stir and cook until it browns.

2. Add vinegar, salt, pepper, stock, tomato paste, cinnamon,

lemon peel, thyme and ghee, stir, cook for 3 minutes and

transfer everything to your slow cooker.

3. Cover and cook on High for 4 hours.

4. Discard cinnamon, lemon peel and thyme, add parsley, stir and

divide into bowls.

5. Serve hot.

Nutrition: cal.250, fat 6, fiber 1, carbs 7, protein 33

44. **Pork Stew**

Preparation time: 10 minutes **Cooking time:** 1 hour and 20 minutes **Servings:**

12

Ingredients:

- 2 tbsp. coconut oil
- 4 pounds pork, cubed
- Salt and black pepper to the taste
- 2 tbsp. ghee
- 3 garlic cloves, minced
- ¾ cup beef stock
- ¾ cup apple cider vinegar
- 3 carrots, chopped
- 1 cabbage head, shredded
- ½ cup green onion, chopped
- 1 cup whipping cream

Instructions:

1. Heat up a pan with the ghee and the oil over medium high heat,

add pork and brown it for a few minutes on each side.

2. Add vinegar and stock, stir well and bring to a simmer.

3. Add cabbage, garlic, salt and pepper, stir, cover and cook for 1

hour.

4. Add carrots and green onions, stir and cook for 15 minutes more.

5. Add whipping cream, stir for 1 minute, divide between plates and serve.

Nutrition: cal.400, fat 25, fiber 3, carbs 6, protein 43

45. <u>Sausage Stew</u>

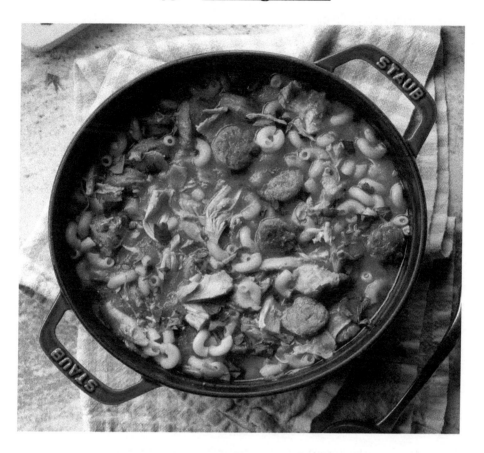

Preparation time: 10 minutes **Cooking time:** 20 minutes **Servings:** 9

Ingredients:

- 1 pound smoked sausage, sliced
- 1 green bell pepper, chopped
- 2 yellow onions, chopped
- Salt and black pepper to the taste
- 1 cup parsley, chopped

- 8 green onions, chopped
- ¼ cup avocado oil
- 1 cup beef stock
- 6 garlic cloves
- 28 ounces canned tomatoes, chopped
- 16 ounces okra, chopped
- 8 ounces tomato sauce
- 2 tbsp. coconut aminos
- 1 tbsp. gluten free hot sauce

Instructions:

1. Heat up a pot with the oil over medium high heat, add

sausages, stir and cook for 2 minutes.

2. Add onion, bell pepper, green onions, parsley, salt and pepper,

stir and cook for 2 minutes more.

3. Add stock, garlic, tomatoes, okra, tomato sauce, coconut

aminos and hot sauce, stir, bring to a simmer and cook for 15

minutes.

4. Add more salt and pepper, stir, divide into bowls and serve.

Nutrition: cal.274, fat 20, fiber 4, carbs 7, protein 10

46. **Burgundy Beef Stew**

Preparation time: 10 minutes **Cooking time:** 3 hours **Servings:** 7

Ingredients:

- 2 pounds beef chuck roast, cubed
- 15 ounces canned tomatoes, chopped
- 4 carrots, chopped
- Salt and black pepper to the taste
- ½ pounds mushrooms, sliced
- 2 celery ribs, chopped
- 2 yellow onions, chopped
- 1 cup beef stock
- 1 tbsp. thyme, chopped
- ½ tsp. mustard powder
- 3 tbsp. almond flour
- 1 cup water

Instructions:

1. Heat up an oven proof pot over medium high heat, add beef

cubes, stir and brown them for a couple of minutes on each

side.

2. Add tomatoes, mushrooms, onions, carrots, celery, salt, pepper

mustard, stock and thyme and stir.

3. In a bowl mix water with flour and stir well.

Add this to the pot, stir well, introduce in the oven and bake at

325 degrees F for 3 hours.

4. Stir every half an hour.

5. Divide into bowls and serve.

Nutrition: cal.275, fat 13, fiber 4, carbs 7, protein 28

Vegetable Recipes

47. <u>**Arugula And Broccoli Soup**</u>

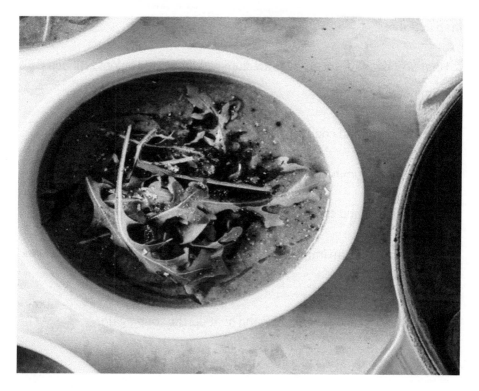

Preparation time: 10 minutes **Cooking time:** 20 minutes **Servings:** 4

Ingredients:

- 1 small yellow onion, chopped
- 1 tbsp. olive oil
- 1 garlic clove, minced
- 1 broccoli head, florets separated
- Salt and black pepper to the taste
- 2 and ½ cups veggie stock

- 1 tsp. cumin, ground
- Juice of ½ lemon
- 1 cup arugula leaves

Instructions:

1. Heat up a pot with the oil over medium high heat, add onions, stir and cook for 4 minutes.

2. Add garlic, stir and cook for 1 minute.

3. Add broccoli, cumin, salt and pepper, stir and cook for 4 minutes.

4. Add stock, stir and cook for 8 minutes.

5. Blend soup using an immersion blender, add half of the arugula and blend again.

6. Add the rest of the arugula, stir and heat up the soup again.

7. Add lemon juice, stir, ladle into soup bowls and serve.

Nutrition: cal. 150, fat 3, fiber 1, carbs 3, protein 7

48. <u>Zucchini Cream</u>

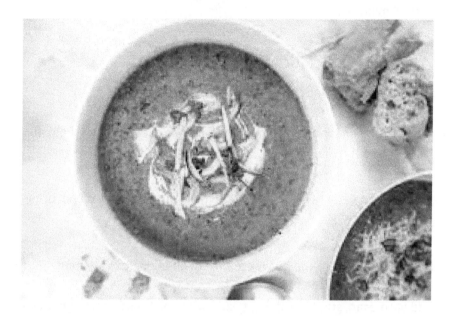

Preparation time: 10 minutes **Cooking time:** 25 minutes **Servings:** 8

Ingredients:

- 6 zucchinis, cut in halves and then sliced
- Salt and black pepper to the taste
- 1 tbsp. ghee
- 28 ounces veggie stock
- 1 tsp. oregano, dried
- ½ cup yellow onion, chopped
- 3 garlic cloves, minced
- 2 ounces parmesan, grated
- ¾ cup heavy cream

Instructions:

1. Heat up a pot with the ghee over medium high heat, add onion, stir and cook for 4 minutes.

2. Add garlic, stir and cook for 2 minutes more.

3. Add zucchinis, stir and cook for 3 minutes.

4. Add stock, stir, bring to a boil and simmer over medium heat for 15 minutes.

5. Add oregano, salt and pepper, stir, take off heat and blend using an immersion blender.

6. Heat up soup again, add heavy cream, stir and bring to a simmer.

7. Add parmesan, stir, take off heat, ladle into bowls and serve right away.

Nutrition: cal.160, fat 4, fiber 2, carbs 4, protein 8

49. Zucchini And Avocado Soup

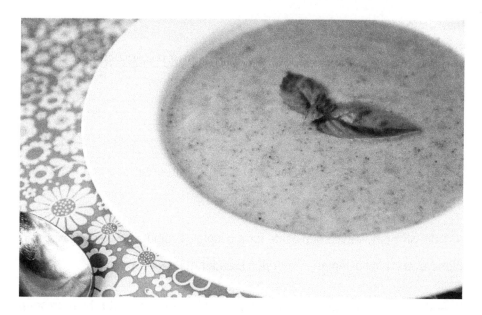

Preparation time: 10 minutes **Cooking time:** 15 minutes **Servings:** 4

Ingredients:

- 1 big avocado, pitted, peeled and chopped
- 4 scallions, chopped
- 1 tsp. ginger, grated
- 2 tbsp. avocado oil
- Salt and black pepper to the taste
- 2 zucchinis, chopped
- 29 ounces veggie stock
- 1 garlic clove, minced
- 1 cup water
- 1 tbsp. lemon juice

- 1 red bell pepper, chopped

Instructions:

1. Heat up a pot with the oil over medium heat, add onions, stir and cook for 3 minutes.

2. Add garlic and ginger, stir and cook for 1 minute.

3. Add zucchini, salt, pepper, water and stock, stir, bring to a boil, cover pot and cook for 10 minutes.

4. Take off heat, leave soup aside for a couple of minutes, add avocado, stir, blend everything using an immersion blender and heat up again.

5. Add more salt and pepper, bell pepper and lemon juice, stir, heat up soup again, ladle into soup bowls and serve.

Nutrition: cal.154, fat 12, fiber 3, carbs 5, protein 4

50. Swiss Chard Pie

Preparation time: 10 minutes **Cooking time:** 45 minutes **Servings:** 12

Ingredients:

- 8 cups Swiss chard, chopped
- ½ cup onion, chopped
- 1 tbsp. olive oil
- 1 garlic clove, minced
- Salt and black pepper to the taste
- 3 eggs
- 2 cups ricotta cheese
- 1 cup mozzarella, shredded
- A pinch of nutmeg
- ¼ cup parmesan, grated
- 1 pound sausage, chopped

Instructions:

1. Heat up a pan with the oil over medium heat, add onions and garlic, stir and cook for 3 minutes.

2. Add Swiss chard, stir and cook for 5 minutes more.

3. Add salt, pepper and nutmeg, stir, take off heat and leave aside for a few minutes.

4. In a bowl, whisk eggs with mozzarella, parmesan and ricotta and stir well.

5. Add Swiss chard mix and stir well.

6. Spread sausage meat on the bottom of a pie pan and press well.

7. Add Swiss chard and eggs mix, spread well, introduce in the oven at 350 degrees F and bake for 35 minutes.

8. Leave pie aside to cool down, slice and serve it.

Nutrition: cal.332, fat 23, fiber 3, carbs 4, protein 23

51. <u>Swiss Chard Salad</u>

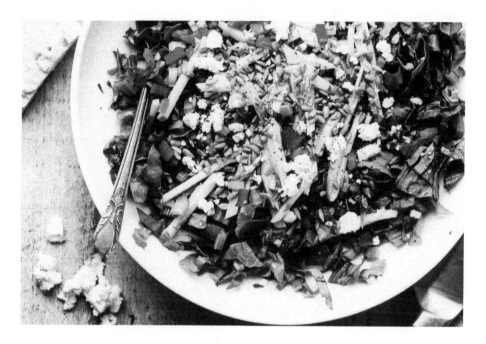

Preparation time: 10 minutes **Cooking time:** 20 minutes **Servings:** 4

Ingredients:

- 1 bunch Swiss chard, cut into strips
- 2 tbsp. avocado oil
- 1 small yellow onion, chopped
- A pinch of red pepper flakes
- ¼ cup pine nuts, toasted
- ¼ cup raisins
- 1 tbsp. balsamic vinegar
- Salt and black pepper to the taste

Instructions:

1. Heat up a pan with the oil over medium heat, add chard and onions, stir and cook for 5 minutes.

2. Add salt, pepper and pepper flakes, stir and cook for 3 minutes more.

3. Put raisins in a bowl, add water to cover them, heat them up in your microwave for 1 minute, leave aside for 5 minutes and drain them well.

4. Add raisins and pine nuts to the pan, also add vinegar, stir, cook for 3 minutes more, divide between plates and serve.

Nutrition: cal. 120, fat 2, fiber 1, carbs 4, protein 8

52. **Green Salad**

Preparation time: 10 minutes **Cooking time:** 0 minutes **Servings:** 4

Ingredients:

- 4 handfuls grapes, halved
- 1 bunch Swiss chard, chopped
- 1 avocado, pitted, peeled and cubed
- Salt and black pepper to the taste
- 2 tbsp. avocado oil
- 1 tbsp. mustard
- 7 sage leaves, chopped
- 1 garlic clove, minced

Instructions:

1. In a salad bowl, mix Swiss chard with grapes and avocado cubes.

2. In a bowl, mix mustard with oil, sage, garlic, salt and pepper and whisk well.

3. Add this to salad, toss to coat well and serve.

Nutrition: cal. 120, fat 2, fiber 1, carbs 4, protein 5

53. Catalan Style Greens

Preparation time: 10 minutes **Cooking time:** 15 minutes **Servings:** 4

Ingredients:

- 1 apple, cored and chopped
- 1 yellow onion, sliced
- 3 tbsp. avocado oil
- ¼ cup raisins
- 6 garlic cloves, chopped
- ¼ cup pine nuts, toasted
- ¼ cup balsamic vinegar
- 5 cups mixed spinach and chard
- Salt and black pepper to the taste
- A pinch of nutmeg

Instructions:

1. Heat up a pan with the oil over medium high heat, add onion, stir and cook for 3 minutes.

2. Add apple, stir and cook for 4 minutes more.

3. Add garlic, stir and cook for 1 minute.

4. Add raisins, vinegar and mixed spinach and chard, stir and cook for 5 minutes.

5. Add nutmeg, salt and pepper, stir, cook for a few seconds more, divide between plates and serve.

Nutrition: cal.120, fat 1, fiber 2, carbs 3, protein 6

Dessert and Snacks Recipes

54. <u>Coconut And Strawberry Delight</u>

Preparation time: 10 minutes **Cooking time:** 0 minutes **Servings:** 4

Ingredients:

- 1 and ¾ cups coconut cream
- 2 tsp. granulated stevia
- 1 cup strawberries

Instructions:

1. Put coconut cream in a bowl, add stevia and stir very well

using an immersion blender.

2. Add strawberries, fold them gently into the mix, divide dessert

into glasses and serve them cold.

Nutrition: cal.245, fat 24, fiber 1, carbs 5, protein 4

55. <u>Caramel Custard</u>

Preparation time: 10 minutes **Cooking time:** 30 minutes **Servings:** 2

Ingredients:

- 1 and ½ tsp. caramel extract
- 1 cup water
- 2 ounces cream cheese
- 2 eggs
- 1 and ½ tbsp. swerve
- *For the caramel sauce:*
- 2 tbsp. swerve
- 2 tbsp. ghee
- ¼ tsp. caramel extract

Instructions:

1. In your blender, mix cream cheese with water, 1 and ½ tbsp. swerve, 1 and ½ tsp. caramel extract and eggs and blend well.

2. Pour this into 2 greased ramekins, introduce in the oven at 350 degrees F and bake for 30 minutes.

3. Meanwhile, put the ghee in a pot and heat up over medium heat add ¼ tsp. caramel extract and 2 tbsp. swerve, stir well and cook until everything melts.

4. Pour this over caramel custard, leave everything to cool down and serve.

Nutrition: cal.254, fat 24, fiber 1, carbs 2, protein 8

56. <u>Cookie Dough Balls</u>

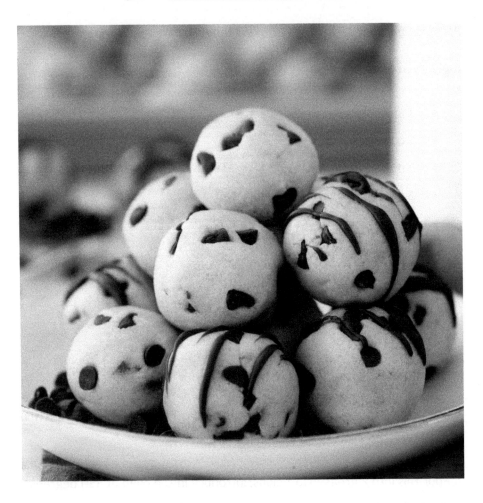

Preparation time: 10 minutes **Servings:** 10

Ingredients:

- ½ cup almond butter
- 3 tbsp. coconut flour
- 3 tbsp. coconut milk
- 1 tsp. cinnamon, powder

- 3 tbsp. coconut sugar
- 15 drops vanilla stevia
- A pinch of salt
- ½ tsp. vanilla extract
- *For the topping:*
- 1 and ½ tsp. cinnamon powder
- 3 tbsp. granulated swerve

Instructions:

1. In a bowl, mix almond butter with 1 tsp. cinnamon, coconut flour, coconut milk, coconut sugar, vanilla extract, vanilla stevia and a pinch of salt and stir well.

2. Shape balls out of this mix.

3. In another bowl mix 1 and ½ tsp. cinnamon powder with swerve and stir well.

4. Roll balls in cinnamon mix and keep them in the fridge until

you serve.

Nutrition: cal.89, fat 1, fiber 2, carbs 4, protein 2

57. **Ricotta Mousse**

Preparation time: 2 hours and 10 minutes **Servings:** 10

Ingredients:

- ½ cup hot coffee
- 2 cups ricotta cheese
- 2 and ½ tsp. gelatin
- 1 tsp. vanilla extract
- 1 tsp. espresso powder
- 1 tsp. vanilla stevia
- A pinch of salt
- 1 cup whipping cream

Instructions:

1. In a bowl, mix coffee with gelatin, stir well and leave aside until coffee is cold.

2. In a bowl, mix espresso, stevia, salt, vanilla extract and ricotta and stir using a mixer.

3. Add coffee mix and stir everything well.

4. Add whipping cream and blend mixture again.

5. Divide into dessert bowls and serve after you've kept it in the fridge for 2 hours.

Nutrition: cal.160, fat 13, fiber 0, carbs 2, protein 7

58. Dessert Granola

Preparation time: 10 minutes **Cooking time:** 35 minutes **Servings:** 4

Ingredients:

- 1 cup coconut, unsweetened and shredded
- 1 cup almonds and pecans, chopped
- 2 tbsp. stevia
- ½ cup pumpkin seeds
- ½ cup sunflower seeds
- 2 tbsp. coconut oil
- 1 tsp. nutmeg, ground
- 1 tsp. apple pie spice mix

Instructions:

1. In a bowl, mix almonds and pecans with pumpkin seeds, sunflower seeds, coconut, nutmeg and apple pie spice mix and stir well.

2. Heat up a pan with the coconut oil over medium heat, add stevia and stir until they combine.

3. Pour this over nuts and coconut mix and stir well.

4. Spread this on a lined baking sheet, introduce in the oven at 300 degrees F and bake for 30 minutes.

5. Leave your granola to cool down, cut and serve it.

Nutrition: cal.120, fat 2, fiber 2, carbs 4, protein 7

59. Peanut Butter And Chia Pudding

Preparation time: 10 minutes **Cooking time:** 0 minutes **Servings:** 4

Ingredients:

- ½ cup chia seeds
- 2 cups almond milk, unsweetened
- 1 tsp. vanilla extract
- ¼ cup peanut butter, unsweetened
- 1 tsp. vanilla stevia
- A pinch of salt

Instructions:

1. In a bowl, mix milk with chia seeds, peanut butter, vanilla extract, stevia and pinch of salt and stir well.

2. Leave this pudding aside for 5 minutes, then stir it again, divide into dessert glasses and leave in the fridge for 10 minutes.

Nutrition: cal. 120, fat 1, fiber 2, carbs 4, protein 2

60. __Pumpkin Custard__

Preparation time: 10 minutes **Cooking time:** 5 minutes **Servings:** 6

Ingredients:

- 1 tbsp. gelatin
- ¼ cup warm water
- 14 ounces canned coconut milk
- 14 ounces canned pumpkin puree
- A pinch of salt
- 2 tsp. vanilla extract
- 1 tsp. cinnamon powder
- 1 tsp. pumpkin pie spice
- 8 scoops stevia
- 3 tbsp. erythritol

Instructions:

1. In a pot, mix pumpkin puree with coconut milk, a pinch of salt,

vanilla extract, cinnamon powder, stevia, erythritol and pumpkin pie spice, stir well and heat up for a couple of minutes.

2. In a bowl, mix gelatin and water and stir.

3. Combine the 2 mixtures, stir well, divide custard into ramekins

and leave aside to cool down.

4. Keep in the fridge until you serve it.

Nutrition: cal. 200, fat 2, fiber 1, carbs 3, protein 5

61. No Bake Cookies

Preparation time: 40 minutes **Cooking time:** 2 minutes **Servings:** 4

Ingredients:

- 1 cup swerve
- ¼ cup coconut milk
- ¼ cup coconut oil
- 2 tbsp. cocoa powder
- 1 and ¾ cup coconut, shredded
- ½ tsp. vanilla extract
- A pinch of salt
- ¾ cup almond butter

Instructions:

1. Heat up a pan with the oil over medium high heat, add milk, cocoa powder and swerve, stir well for about 2 minutes and take off heat.

2. Add vanilla, a pinch of salt, coconut and almond butter and stir very well.

3. Place spoonful of this mix on a lined baking sheet, keep in the fridge for 30 minutes and then serve them.

Nutrition: cal. 150, fat 2, fiber 1, carbs 3, protein 6